SHIATSU MASSAGE MANUAL

Comprehensive Manual To
Understanding The Principles &
Techniques Of Shiatsu Therapy

DEAN OTTO

Contents

Introductory

Japanese shiatsu massage entails putting pressure on certain places all over the body. The Japanese word "shiatsu" means "finger pressure" in English.

Traditional Chinese medicine (TCM) is the theoretical foundation of this massage method. It centers on the idea of qi (or Chi), the life force energy that is thought to circulate throughout the body via channels called meridians.

Rhythmic pressure is applied to different areas along the body's meridians by use of fingers, thumbs, palms, and occasionally elbows or knees during a Shiatsu massage. The objective is to encourage a state of harmony and health by enhancing the flow of Qi. The client stays completely clothed while the shiatsu practitioner works on them on a futon or mat laid out on the floor.

To alleviate stress and promote better energy flow throughout the body, Shiatsu practitioners may use finger pressure, stretches, and joint rotations, among other techniques. As a holistic method, it helps with issues including pain, stress, tension, and imbalances in the body.

It's important to remember that Shiatsu is its own type of bodywork with its own specific methods and approaches, often including parts of Western medicine's anatomy and physiology, even though it has certain similarities with traditional Chinese medicine.

It is recommended that you discuss any health issues with a licensed professional before undergoing a Shiatsu session, as is the case with any type of massage or bodywork.

CHAPTER ONE
Shiatsu Fundamentals

The foundational ideas of shiatsu are rooted in both Japanese and traditional Chinese medicine. Among the many tenets of Shiatsu are the following:

• Qi, also known as Chi, is a fundamental principle of Shiatsu. It is the life force energy that moves through the body via channels called meridians. It is thought that general health and well-being depend on the steady flow of Qi.

• Shiatsu is centered around acupoints and meridians, which are routes for the flow of Qi. Acupoints are pressure sites along these meridians that practitioners use to either balance or promote the flow of Qi.

• The fundamental tenet of Shiatsu is the need of maintaining a state of harmonious balance in the energy field of the client. It is believed that disruptions or imbalances in the flow of Qi can amplify both mental and bodily pain. The goal of shiatsu is to help the body's inherent healing mechanisms and return harmony to the system.

• Shiatsu considers the whole person, including their mind, spirit, and physical self, while assessing their health. By tending to one's mental and emotional health as well as one's physical health, the treatment promotes complete recovery.

• Aside from Qi, the Japanese word "Ki" is frequently utilized in Shiatsu to denote the vital life force or energy. A feeling of vigor and calmness is sought after by the practitioner by increasing the flow of Ki.

• Shiatsu makes use of non-invasive treatments including light stretching, palm pressure, and finger pressure. Fingers, thumbs, palms, elbows, and even knees are used to apply pressure. Without the use of needles or oils, this method is intended to be calming and beneficial.

• Active Client Participation: Shiatsu frequently requires the receiver to take an active role in the treatment. In order to create a more conscious and intimate connection between the therapist and patient, the client may be instructed to take deep breaths, relax, and actively participate in the procedure.

• Shiatsu is not only used to treat symptoms, but also as a preventative measure and to keep the body in good health generally. Maintaining a steady equilibrium and strength in the body may necessitate frequent sessions.

Although these concepts form the basis of Shiatsu, it's worth noting that different practitioners may use different techniques and approaches. Since shiatsu's efficacy varies from patient to patient, it's best to talk to a trained professional about your unique health issues and treatment objectives before beginning treatment.

Ki Principles (Power)

The idea of "Ki" or "Qi" is central to many East Asian traditions, including martial arts, traditional Japanese medicine, and traditional Chinese medicine.

Traditional uses of the phrase may vary in spelling from one culture to another, but the meaning is the same: it describes the vital energy or life force said to permeate all forms of life.

Here are a few important ideas concerning Ki:

• Vital Energy or Ki: Ki is frequently said to be what keeps all living things going. It is believed to permeate every part of nature and constitute the very core of existence.

• A condition of health is considered as one in which the flow of Qi is balanced and harmonious in traditional Chinese medicine and associated activities.

It is thought that imbalances or obstructions in the flow of Ki contribute to sickness or pain. Restoring or maintaining a balanced flow of energy is the goal of practices such as acupuncture, Qi Gong, and Shiatsu.

• There are certain channels or routes in the body called meridians through which the life force energy (Ki) is said to flow. A healthy body relies on a steady flow of Ki along these meridians, which are linked to different systems and organs.

• Integral to the mind-body relationship is the concept of ki. According to traditional belief, one's emotional and mental health affect one's Ki flow, and vice versa, one's emotional and mental health might affect one's Ki balance. It is common practice to build and balance Ki through awareness and meditation.

• The importance of knowing and using Ki in martial arts is emphasized in numerous schools of thought. Some practitioners think that they can improve their physical talents, focus, and martial ability by directing and growing Ki. Words like "hara" in Japanese karate often bring this idea to mind.

• Various activities are developed to improve the flow and balance of Ki. Among these are the Chinese arts of Qi Gong and Tai Chi, the Japanese practices of Reiki and Shiatsu, and the specialized breathing exercises and meditation that are a part of these traditions.

• In traditional medical practices such as acupuncture and acupressure, the central idea is ki, which is used to influence the flow of energy by stimulating certain places on the body. As a Japanese healing technique, Reiki involves the practice of "channeling" energy (Ki) to alleviate stress and speed recovery.

The idea of Ki has its origins in traditional belief systems, therefore people from different cultures and backgrounds may have diverse interpretations of it. Traditional traditions rely heavily on it, although its meaning and acceptability might vary depending on the prevailing philosophical and cultural views.

CHAPTER TWO
Acupuncture And The Meridians

The core idea of acupuncture, acupressure, and traditional Chinese medicine (TCM) is the idea of pressure points and meridians. The following is a synopsis of these ideas:

1. The meridians:

• The body's meridians are channels through which the vital energy, or Qi, flows. A different organ or physiological system is linked to one of the twelve main meridians.

• Pathways: These pathways, which are actually networks of meridians, link the external body to its internal organs. For optimal health and harmony, it is essential that Qi flow along the unique pathways that each meridian follows.

• Health, according to traditional Chinese medicine, is achieved when the meridians are free to move in a balanced and harmonious fashion, a condition known as qi flow. It is believed that a variety of physical and mental health problems can be attributed to disruptions or imbalances in the flow of Qi.

2. Medicinal Pressure Points:

• Acupuncture points, or acupoints, are strategic spots on the body that are believed to have healing properties. The meridians are a common place to find these spots.

• There are a number of methods for stimulating acupoints, including acupuncture (the use of needles), acupressure (the application of pressure using fingers or other tools), cupping, and moxibustion.

• Purposes: There are several benefits and functions linked to each acupoint. According to traditional Chinese medicine, stimulating these sites can influence Qi flow, bring about a state of equilibrium, and alleviate certain health issues.

• For instance, there are a number of well-known acupoints, such as LI4 (Hegu) on the hand, which is said to alleviate pain and headaches, and ST36 (Zusanli) on the lower thigh, which is said to stimulate the immune system and provide energy.

3. Swedish massage:

• The technique of acupressure is to increase the flow of Qi and create balance by applying pressure to certain acupoints on the body.

• Method: Acupressure can be applied using a variety of utensils, including fingers, thumbs, elbows, or specialized equipment. Applying pressure in a rhythmic and methodical fashion is the norm.

• Pain treatment, stress reduction, relaxation, and general well-being are just a few of the many benefits of acupressure. Many people choose to self-administer this method because it is non-invasive.

Based on their understanding of the body's meridians and acupoints, acupuncturists and acupressure practitioners design individualized treatment programs for each patient. Although these notions have their origins in TCM, you may find them in other traditional healing systems like Shiatsu in Japan and Sujok in Korea. While these methods have been around for a while, the effectiveness of complementary and alternative medicine is something that is always being studied and researched.

A Balanced Approach To Shiatsu

Understanding the body's energy balance is central to Shiatsu and TCM, the fields that draw from traditional Chinese medicine. The connection between Shiatsu and Yin and Yang is as follows:

1. Essentials of Yin and Yang:

• The duality character of the universe is symbolized by the core ideas of Yin and Yang in Traditional Chinese Medicine (TCM) philosophy. In fact, they are opposing forces that are dependent on and connected to one another.

• Yin: Yin is linked to attributes like openness, tranquility, shadows, chillyness, and femininity.

• Yang: Masculinity, action, movement, brightness, and heat are all aspects of Yang.

• Harmony: A healthy body and mind are the result of a harmonious relationship between the Yin and Yang forces. People often attribute their health problems to disruptions in these forces.

2. In the Body, Yin and Yang:

• TCM assigns a Yin or Yang energy to each system of the body's organs. As an illustration, the Yang organs are the heart and lungs, whereas the Yin organs are the liver and kidneys.

• The body's meridians are said to possess both yin and yang attributes. The Yin and Yang aspects of certain meridians are more pronounced than those of others.

3. When it comes to Shiatsu,

• Diagnosis: Shiatsu therapists frequently use palpation and careful observation to determine the client's Yin-Yang balance. In doing so, they may seek out indications of an imbalance between the Yin and Yang aspects.

• Shiatsu is a form of alternative medicine that attempts to harmonize the body's Yin and Yang energy. When a person is feeling too much Yang, the practitioner can work on tonifying the Yin energy, and the opposite is also true. If a client is experiencing excessive stress (Yang), a Shiatsu session could focus on grounding and relaxation to improve Yin.

• Practitioners can attain balance through meridian work by selecting acupoints or meridians according to their Yin or Yang energy.

4. Stabilization and Balance:

• Health: Similar to Traditional Chinese Medicine (TCM), Shiatsu aims to improve the equilibrium of the body's Yin and Yang energies. The body is seen to be at its most healthy state when these energies are balanced.

• Prevention: Shiatsu isn't just for when you're sick; it can also help keep the Yin and Yang energies balanced and stop imbalances from manifesting in the first place.

One of the most important things you can learn about Shiatsu is how to balance and harmonize your body's Yin and Yang energies. As a result, practitioners are better able to adapt their methods to the specific needs of their patients.

CHAPTER THREE
The Art Of Shiatsu Massage Preparation

To make sure you have a pleasant and productive Shiatsu massage, there are a few things to think about before you go in. In general, these are the rules:

1. Expressing ideas:

• Health Details: Communicate any pertinent medical history, injuries, or concerns to your Shiatsu practitioner. With this data, the therapist can better meet your individual requirements throughout the session.

2. What to Wear:

• Loose, comfortable clothes is recommended. Because shiatsu is most effective when the client is fully clothed, it's important to wear loose-fitting clothing so the therapist may move freely around in. Stay away from belts and other tight accessories.

3. Nutrition and Fluids:

• To keep pain at bay during your Shiatsu session, it's best to avoid eating a large meal in the hours leading up to it.

• Raise your water intake to ensure you're properly hydrated before your activity.

4. Time of Arrival:

• Get There Early: Don't be tardy for your appointment; that way, you'll have plenty of time to fill out any paperwork or address any concerns you may have with your practitioner.

5. Calming Down:

• Practice attentive breathing for a few minutes before the session. Take a few deep breaths to calm down and get ready for the massage.

6. Outline Your Goals:

• Talk to your Shiatsu practitioner about your preferences in pressure and techniques, as well as any particular places you'd like them to concentrate on.

7. Keep Your Mind Open:

• Keep the lines of communication open with your practitioner during the session. Make sure them know if the pressure is too much or if you're uncomfortable. Similarly, please do not hesitate to express any preferences or detailed criticisms you may have.

8. After The Massage:

• Hydrate: To aid in the elimination of any toxins generated during the massage, drink water after the session.

• Wind Down: After the workout, give yourself a chance to relax and unwind if at all feasible. It is best to refrain from exerting yourself too soon following.

9. Additional Suggestions:

• Home Remedies: To help you get the most out of your Shiatsu massage, your therapist may suggest some self-care measures, such stretching, exercises, or changes to your daily routine.

Keep in mind the importance of communicating. Feel free to communicate with your Shiatsu practitioner any worries, inquiries, or personal preferences you may have. On top of that, because you are an individual, your preparation may differ according to your personal tastes and health requirements.

Fundamental Shiatsu Methods

In shiatsu, acupressure is used to alleviate stress, restore harmony to the body's energy channels, and treat a wide range of mental and physical ailments. Despite the complexity and skill required for the practice, below are some of the more fundamental Shiatsu techniques you may come across:

1. Practices in Palming and Finger Pressure:

• The practitioner may exert wide, even pressure over bigger sections of the body using the palms of their hands.

• Applying targeted pressure to acupoints or regions of tension might be done with fingers, thumbs, or particular portions of the hand.

2. Working the Muscles:

• Kneading: This is accomplished by lifting and gently squeezing the muscles with the palms and fingers, much as when you knead dough.

• Tapping: To ease muscles and promote energy flow, one may utilize light tapping or rhythmic drumming motions.

3. Rotations and Stretching:

• Gentle stretching movements can be used to alleviate stress and increase range of motion.

• Passive rotations of the joints may be performed by practitioners to promote relaxation and increased mobility.

4. Navigation by Palm and Thumb:

• The practitioner applies pressure along the meridians or specific parts of the body by strolling with their palms.

• Thumb walking: it's like palm walking, but you focus on acupoints or muscle knots with your thumbs.

5. Pressure within the blood vessels:

• Pressure applied in circular motions, typically with the thumbs or palms, can aid in the release of stress and the promotion of circulation.

6. Supporting and swaying:

• Holding: To promote energy flow or resolve particular problems, the practitioner could just hold pressure on specific spots.

• Relaxation and the body's own healing processes can be enhanced through rhythmic motions or light rocking.

7. Mindfulness of Breath:

• Guided Breathing: To help clients relax and increase energy flow, practitioners may suggest deep, mindful breathing exercises during the session.

8. Tracing the Meridians:

• Meridian Lines: Pressing on acupoints while one moves along the routes of certain meridians is one such technique.

Remember that Shiatsu is usually done when the client is fully clothed. Adjusting the pressure according to the individual's tastes and demands, the techniques are applied to produce balance and relaxation.

Furthermore, Shiatsu takes into account not just the physical but also the mental, emotional, and energy components of health. Getting Shiatsu from a professional is the best way to ensure a safe and productive session.

CHAPTER FOUR
Comprehensive Shiatsu Program

You need to know all the ins and outs of Shiatsu to do a full-body Shiatsu session. An overview of the body's major systems is provided here.

The client's preferences and any particular health concerns should inform the adjustment of the applied pressure; this is only a basic guide. It is recommended that you consult an expert if you are not already trained in Shiatsu.

1. Begin by centering:

• Start by taking a few deep breaths and centering yourself, as well as the client.

• Get to know each other and decide what you want to accomplish during the session.

2. Shoulders and Neck:

• Press down on the shoulders and neck using your palms and fingers.

• To relieve stress, knead the area or roll it in a circle.

• Be sure to incorporate light rotations and stretches.

3. In the past:

• Use palm walking or thumb pressure to work along the spine.

• Firmly press down on the muscles that support your back in a circular motion.

• Gently stretch while kneading.

4. Physical Dexterity:

• Use your palms and fingers to provide pressure on your arms and hands.

• Be sure to incorporate finger and wrist stretches.

• The acupoints on the arms should be carefully considered.

5. Foot and Leg:

• Using circular motions, thumb pressures, and palm walking, strengthen your legs.

• Stretch the legs, specifically the ankles and knees.

• Keep your attention on your feet while you walk in a circular pattern with your thumbs.

• Focus on the foot and leg acupoints.

6. Lower body:

• Apply light, circular pressure on the abdomen in a clockwise motion, mirroring the body's natural digestive process.

• Be careful not to apply too much pressure if the client is experiencing gastrointestinal problems or pain.

7. Head and Face:

• Focus on the acupoints on your face and gently push them with your palms and fingers.

• Make small, circular strokes over your scalp.

- Consider massaging the client's jaw and ears if they feel comfortable with it.

- Start with a heavier touch and gradually ease off.

- Allow the client to assimilate the session by offering a few moments of stillness.

- Make sure to mention any aftercare instructions, like to stay hydrated.

Staying present, paying close attention to the client's body language, and being flexible are the three most important aspects of a good Shiatsu session.

Furthermore, it is crucial to see an expert before trying to do a full-body Shiatsu program if you are not already a skilled Shiatsu practitioner.

Pregnancy And Shiatsu

Shiatsu can be modified to offer pregnant women a gentle and comforting form of treatment. Nevertheless, it is essential to exercise caution when practicing prenatal Shiatsu and to get the advice of a healthcare professional before to engaging in any form of massage therapy while pregnant.

Some things to think about while deciding to use Shiatsu during pregnancy are:

1. Advice from a Medical Professional:

• It is important for pregnant women to talk to their doctor before getting a massage of any kind, especially Shiatsu, to make sure it won't harm them.

2. Skilled Professional:

• Locate a Shiatsu practitioner who has prior expertise treating expectant mothers. To make sure the mother-to-be is safe and comfortable, certain adjustments are required, and not all massage therapists have received prenatal massage training.

3. Setting the Stage:

• Make sure the pregnant person is in a comfortable position throughout the session. To alleviate strain on the abdomen, it is generally advised to lie on one's side or slightly recline, particularly in the latter weeks of pregnancy.

4. Changes and Things to Stay Away From:

• When you're expecting a child, it's best to stay away from acupressure sites and procedures that can cause your uterus to contract.

• We can highlight gentle, supportive strategies that help with relaxation and common pregnant pains.

5. Maximize Your Comfort:

• Instead of deep tissue work, sessions should center around making you feel comfortable and relaxed.

• Pressure should be adjusted according to the person's comfort level, taking care not to apply too much pressure to sensitive places.

6. Key Focus Areas:

• Shiatsu can alleviate some of the pain and swelling that some pregnant women experience in particular locations, including the lower back, hips, and ankles.

• To improve flexibility and alleviate stress, you might use light stretches and joint mobilizations.

7. Mindfulness of Breath:

• Make use of breathing exercises to help you relax and reduce stress.

8. Drinking enough water:

• Expectant mothers should be reminded to drink water before and after the session because staying hydrated is crucial for their health.

9. Suggestions for Continued Care:

• Suggest ways to care for yourself after the treatment, like doing self-massages at home, being physically active, and drinking enough of water.

10. Expressing ideas:

• The practitioner and client must have an open line of communication. The practitioner should modify their tactics based on the client's expressed discomfort or worries.

The health of the mother and child should take precedence throughout pregnancy because of the special and delicate nature of the time. Before contemplating massage therapy while pregnant, it is important to check with a healthcare expert and choose a trained and experienced Shiatsu practitioner.

CHAPTER FIVE
Child-Friendly Shiatsu

Children can benefit from shiatsu in a variety of ways, including a gentle and non-invasive technique that promotes physical and mental health. Careful consideration of the child's developmental stage and unique demands is essential when administering Shiatsu to children. Some things to think about are:

1. Experienced Professional:

• If you are looking for a Shiatsu practitioner who has experience with children, it is crucial to find one for your child. They ought to be adept at adjusting their methods based on what they learn about children's growth and development.

2. Parental Permission and Participation:

• Before giving Shiatsu to a child, make sure to get their parents' permission.

• For the sake of the child's comfort and trust, parents may choose to accompany their younger children during the session.

3. More Concise Meetings:

• Sessions with children are often shorter than with adults because their attention spans are likely to be shorter. Sessions lasting 15 to 30 minutes can be better suited for kids.

4. Optimistic Perspective:

• To make the experience fun for the kid, add a playful and engaging touch.

• Keep the language and methods engaging and suitable for the age group.

5. What to Wear:

• Young ones can benefit from Shiatsu while fully clothed. Make sure they are wearing comfortable clothing, and modify the training accordingly.

6. Soft Caress:

• Shiatsu for kids typically uses less pressure than sessions for adults.

• Relax and increase energy flow with a little touch.

7. Link Between Mind and Body:

• Do age-appropriate mindfulness or breath-awareness exercises with the child.

• Motivate the youngster to join in whatever they feel most at ease.

8. Points of Interest:

• Shiatsu is a great way to help kids who are dealing with stress, growing pains, or muscle strain.

• Practice certain regions, such as the feet, shoulders, and back, by adjusting your techniques.

9. Deference to Personal Space:

• Pay attention to the child's limits and how they feel comfortable. On every session, make sure to ask for their feedback.

10. Parental Education and Engagement:

• Inform parents of the positive effects of Shiatsu on children and giving them easy ways to incorporate the practice into their daily routine to help their child feel better.

11. Ability to Modify:

• Respond quickly and adjust your behavior based on what the youngster needs. A more energetic method may work better for some kids, while a more relaxing one may be more their speed.

Before contemplating any type of bodywork on a child, be sure their comfort and safety your top priority. Before introducing Shiatsu or any other complementary therapy to a kid, it is important to check with a healthcare provider if there are any health issues or if the child is receiving medical treatment.

Shiatsu For The Aged

Shiatsu, a gentle and effective therapy that can help the elderly in many ways, both physically and emotionally, is becoming more popular. Nevertheless, when providing Shiatsu to the elderly, it is crucial to take into account their unique health concerns, mobility limitations, and comfort levels. Some things to think about are:

1. Medical Evaluation:

• It's crucial to perform a comprehensive health evaluation before administering Shiatsu to an elderly person. Take into account any current health difficulties, prescriptions, and mobility concerns.

2. Expressing ideas:

• Get to know the elderly person's level of comfort, their preferences, and any worries they might have by establishing open lines of communication.

3. Appropriate Posture:

• Always put the old person in a position where they will be most comfortable. Chairs, massage tables, or even the patient's bed can all be used for Shiatsu treatments, depending on the patient's movement needs.

4. Soft Methods:

• If the person is more susceptible to bruising, has thin muscles, or sensitive skin, be extra careful and use modified approaches.

• Change the amount of pressure till it feels right for the individual.

5. Mobility of the Joints:

• To increase flexibility, try including light joint rotations and stretches, paying special attention to the hips, knees, and shoulders, which are areas that tend to get stiff.

6. Coziness and Heat:

• To make sure the old person is comfortable during the session, make sure the environment is warm and utilize blankets or other coverings.

7. Address Particular Concerns:

• Take on certain problems that many seniors have, like aches and pains, poor blood flow, or tight muscles.

• Modify methods to focus on certain regions while taking into account the person's level of comfort.

8. Link Between Mind and Body:

• Combine practices of relaxation and mindfulness. In order to alleviate tension and promote relaxation, it is recommended to breathe slowly and deeply.

9. Drinking enough water:

• It is recommended to drink plenty of water before and after the massage to assist eliminates any toxins that may have been generated.

10. Time management:

• Pay attention to how quickly the session is going. To avoid exhaustion, it's best to keep sessions brief and focused so the patient can be comfortable.

11. Knowing Your Posture:

• Take a stand against poor posture, a prevalent problem in the elderly.

To alleviate pain and promote better posture, try these techniques.

12. Keep Caregivers Informed and Involved:

• Participate in the session with family or caregivers if possible. Give them some basic Shiatsu techniques and teach them how to help an elderly loved one at home.

The care and security of the elderly should always come first. Prior to adopting Shiatsu or any other form of complementary therapy, individuals should seek advice from their healthcare professional regarding any particular health concerns or medications they may be using. Each person's specific needs can be met during a Shiatsu session by a trained and experienced practitioner who is skilled with working with the elderly.

CHAPTER SIX
Dealing With Regular Health Issues

Shiatsu can be customized to address a wide range of common health issues by utilizing targeted techniques on specific acupoints and meridians.

The practice of Shiatsu should not be considered a replacement for traditional medical care, but it has the potential to enhance health in addition to it. The following are examples of typical health issues and possible Shiatsu treatments.

1. **Anxiety and Stress:**

• Methods: Relaxing stretches, deep breathing exercises, and light finger and palm pressure on designated areas.

• Pay close attention to the central meridians, especially those that pass through the heart and the pericardium.

2. **Soreness and Tense Muscles:**

• Massage methods include kneading, applying circular pressure, and stretching to alleviate muscle tension.

• Concentrate on: Applying pressure to specific acupoints along the afflicted meridians and places of discomfort or stress.

3. Migraines & Headaches:

• Approach: A combination of light stretching and pressure on certain areas surrounding the neck, shoulders, and head.

• Highlight: The meridian that runs through the gallbladder, as well as the points surrounding the neck and temples.

4. Disruptions to Sleep and Insomnia:

• Methods: Grounding and calming approaches, with a focus on aspects having to do with controlling one's sleep.

• Pay attention to the meridian systems of the heart, liver, and kidneys; these systems are linked to how you sleep.

5. Pain in the Digestive System:

• Methods: Applying circular pressure to the belly, with an emphasis on digestion-related acupoints.

• Pay attention to the locations on the abdomen and the meridians of the stomach and spleen.

6. Feeling Weak and Tired:

• Methods: Light pressure applied to energy and vitality acupoints, accompanied with revitalizing stretches.

• The Kidney and Spleen meridians should be your primary focus because of their connections to vitality and food.

7. Aches and stiffness in the joints:

• Methods: Rotating the joints, mild stretching, and applying circular pressure to the afflicted joints.

• Pay attention to the important meridian pathways that lead to the afflicted joints.

8. Managing Period Pain and Premenstrual Syndrome:

• Methods: Subtle belly massage and pressure on reproductive-related acupoints.

• The meridian systems of the kidneys, liver, and spleen are important for maintaining a healthy menstrual cycle.

9. Airway Disorders (such as Asthma and Allergies):

• Methods: light chest opening stretches, acupressure sites connected to the lungs, and deep breathing exercises.

• Concentrate on: Acupressure points on the back and chest, the large intestine and lung meridians.

10. Mental and Spiritual Health:

• The methods include acupressure sites linked to emotional

equilibrium as well as grounding and calming strategies.

• Concentrate on the meridian systems of the heart, pericardium, and kidneys; these areas are associated with mental and emotional health.

While Shiatsu can help alleviate certain symptoms and provide emotional support, anyone experiencing severe pain should see a doctor for a proper diagnosis and course of therapy.

Furthermore, in order to apply techniques safely and effectively according to the individual's health and preferences, it is recommended to get assistance from a competent Shiatsu practitioner.

Methods For Self-Shimatsu

Although most people get their Shiatsu treatments from certified professionals, there are a few self-Shiatsu techniques that anybody can perform for relaxation and self-care. In most cases, you can do these methods in the comfort of your own home.

Although self-Shiatsu sessions may not be as thorough or precise as those with a professional, they can still be beneficial.

Listed below are several self-Shiatsu methods:

1. Mindfulness of Breath:

• To calm yourself, begin by taking a few minutes to focus on your breathing. Concentrate on taking slow, deep breaths in and out.

2. Release of the Neck and Shoulders:

• In a gentle, circular motion, press down on your skull, neck, and shoulders with your fingertips or thumbs. Reduce stress by doing this.

3. Relieving Headaches:

• Use a circular motion with your thumbs to apply pressure to the acupoints at the temples. For headache relief, this may work.

4. Harmonious Heart Chakra:

• Feel for the intersection of your little and ring fingers on your palm; this is the Heart Meridian. Gently rub in a circular pattern. As a result, you may feel less anxious and more relaxed.

5. Aid for the Digestive System and Stomach:

• To aid digestion, gently press the acupoint two finger widths below the knee cap's centerline. For both legs, make circular motions.

6. Stimulating the Back and Spine:

• While seated, apply pressure and rub along the spine using your fingertips or knuckles, starting at the base and working your way up. By doing so, you can encourage the flow of energy along your back.

7. Shoulder and Lung Support:

• To promote healthy breathing, lightly press with your fingertips along the sides of your rib cage and sternum. A more open chest area may result from this.

8. Muscle Relaxation:

• To ease stress and aid digestion, gently roll your hands over your belly. People who are having trouble digesting food may find this especially useful.

9. The Role of the Foot in Rehabilitation:

• Use your thumbs to press down on certain areas of your feet. Pay close attention to the spots that represent various bodily systems or organs.

10. Maintaining a Healthy Kidney Zone:

• The point on the bottom of your foot that lies between the ball and the arch is the Kidney meridian. Balance can be improved by applying light pressure in circular motions.

Always be mindful to listen to your body and use light touch when practicing self-Shiatsu. It is recommended that you seek the advice of a healthcare professional before engaging in self-Shiatsu if you have any prior health issues. Furthermore, a more thorough and personalized experience can be provided by receiving professional Shiatsu from a trained practitioner.

CHAPTER SEVEN
Mastering The Art Of Shiatsu

A more thorough familiarity with meridian theory, advanced Shiatsu techniques, and the principles of traditional Chinese medicine is required for advanced Shiatsu practices. These techniques are usually only performed by highly trained Shiatsu professionals. Presenting the following advanced Shiatsu techniques:

1. The Five-Element Model:

• In their evaluations and treatments, advanced practitioners frequently incorporate the Five-Element theory. The five elements of this theory—Water, Fire, Earth, and Metal—are correlated with particular organs, meridians, and attributes.

2. Identifying Hara:

• One diagnostic tool in advanced Shiatsu is the hara, or abdominal area. By analyzing the hara, practitioners can learn about their clients' general health and spot any imbalances.

3. Identifying the Pulse:

• Pulse diagnosis is a method that uses the characteristics of the pulse at different wrist locations to determine the health of the organs and meridians. A keen awareness of pulse characteristics and heightened sensitivity are necessary for this task.

4. Elevated Meridian Techniques:

• In order to stimulate and balance energy along particular meridians, more complex and specialized techniques may be employed by advanced practitioners. Techniques such as stretches, joint mobilizations, and targeted acupressure may be part of this.

5. Integrating Emotions and Minds:

• The relationship between emotional and psychological states and physical symptoms is a common area of investigation for advanced Shiatsu practitioners. To improve mental health and correct emotional imbalances, they may use certain methods.

6. The Integration of Movement with Qi Gong: B

• It is an advanced practice to incorporate Qi Gong exercises and movement into Shiatsu sessions. A part of this may include showing clients how to perform certain movements in order to improve their health and the flow of Qi.

7. Balancing the Element of Yang:

• Professionals aim to harmonize the Yin and Yang energies in their bodies, minds, and spirits. This might entail tailoring methods to either calm or stimulate the client's Yin or Yang energies, depending on their preferences.

8. Highly Attuned to Energy and Intuition:

• Many people who practice this art for a long time report feeling more sensitive to energy and intuition.

They may be able to detect when the client's energy field is off and then employ subtle methods to restore harmony.

9. Shiatsu for Trauma:

• Specialists in trauma-informed Shiatsu are able to identify the physical effects of trauma and employ strategies to aid in recovery and resiliency.

10. Combination with Other Approaches:

• To offer a more all-encompassing approach to health and wellness, advanced Shiatsu practitioners may combine their knowledge with aromatherapy, herbal medicine, energy healing, and other healing modalities.

Note that advanced Shiatsu techniques necessitate a strong dedication to the tenets of TCM, as well as substantial training and continuous education in the field. People looking for advanced Shiatsu should look for therapists who have been practicing for a while and have a strong academic background.

Summary

Shiatsu is an integrative form of therapeutic bodywork with its origins in TCM. The goal is to restore harmony to the body's Qi (life force energy) flow through the use of pressure and light stretching. By releasing restrictions and restoring harmony in the body's energy channels, shiatsu can improve one's psychological, physiological, and social health.

The Yin and Yang principles, the interdependence of the body, mind, and spirit, and the knowledge of acupoints and meridians are essential to Shiatsu.

In order to apply pressure to certain points and areas of the body, practitioners often use their hands, fingers, palms, elbows, or knees. Shiatsu can be modified to accommodate different demographics, such as those who are expecting a child, young children, or the elderly.

Fundamental to Shiatsu are the concepts of harmony and balance as well as the body's inherent recuperative powers. Stress, pain, gastrointestinal problems, and emotional imbalances are just some of the many health issues that it is commonly used to treat.

In most cases, shiatsu won't do any harm, but those who are already dealing with specific health issues should talk to their doctor first.

For a more all-encompassing strategy to health and wellbeing, Shiatsu can be mixed with other complementary therapies like acupuncture, massage, yoga, and mindfulness practices.

A more advanced practitioner may also include Qi Gong or movement exercises into their sessions, as well as diagnostic tools such as hara and pulse diagnosis. They may also delve into the Five Element theory.

Shiatsu provides a soothing and all-encompassing way to aid the body's innate recuperative abilities, whether administered by a professional or used as a form of self-care.

To make sure their Shiatsu sessions are safe and effective for them, individuals should seek out the advice of trained professionals if they are interested in trying it out or adding it to their wellness routine.

THE END